Originally from the United States, Dr Jordan now works within the National Health Service in Britain, and specializes in the diseases of the blood. She is a Registrar in a large city hospital and is currently doing research into lifestyles and hypertension. She also has a private clinic where she successfully dispenses advice and treatment in many areas, as well as hypertension.

CONTROLLING YOUR BLOOD PRESSURE

Dr Mary-Beth Jordan

CONTROLLING YOUR BLOOD PRESSURE

Hypertension: Symptoms and Treatment

EMMA
STERN
PUBLISHING

An Emma Stern Publication

A CIP catalogue record for this title is available from the British Library.

ISBN: 978-1-911224-11-2

Published in 2016

Emma Stern Publishing
107 Fleet Street
London
EC4A 2AB

www.emmastern.com
www.facebook.com/emmasternpublishing
Email: editorial@emmastern.com
Email: marketing@emmastern.com

Printed in Great Britain

Hypertension

Hypertension or high blood pressure, sometimes called arterial hypertension, is a chronic medical condition in which the blood pressure in the arteries is elevated.

Blood pressure is summarised by two measurements, systolic and diastolic, which depend on whether the heart muscle is contracting (systole) or relaxed between beats (diastole). This equals the maximum and minimum pressure, respectively.

Normal blood pressure at rest is within the range of 100–140mmHg systolic (top reading) and 60–90mmHg diastolic (bottom reading). High blood pressure is said to be present if it is often at or above 140/90mmHg.

Hypertension is classified as either primary or secondary hypertension; about 90–95% of cases are categorized as primary hypertension which means high blood pressure with no obvious underlying medical cause. The remaining 5–10% of cases (secondary hypertension) are caused by other conditions that affect the kidneys, arteries, heart or endocrine system.

If not treated, hypertension puts strain on the heart, leading to heart disease and coronary artery disease.

Hypertension is also a major risk factor for stroke and kidney disease. A moderately high arterial blood pressure is associated with a shortened life expectancy while mild elevation is not. Dietary and lifestyle changes can improve blood pressure control and decrease the risk of health complications, although drug treatment is still often necessary in some people.

Signs and symptoms

Hypertension is rarely accompanied by any symptoms, and its identification is usually through screening, or when seeking healthcare for an unrelated problem. A proportion of people with high blood pressure report headaches (particularly at the back of the head and usually fiercest in the morning), as well as lightheadedness, vertigo (dizziness) tinnitus (buzzing or hissing in the ears), altered vision or fainting episodes. These symptoms, might, however, be related to anxiety rather than the high blood pressure itself.

Secondary hypertension

Some additional signs and symptoms may suggest secondary hypertension, i.e. hypertension due to an identifiable cause such as kidney diseases or endocrine diseases. For example, obesity, glucose intolerance, and purple stretch marks suggest hypertension.

Hypertensive crisis

Severely elevated blood pressure (equal to or greater than a systolic 180 or diastolic of 110—(sometimes termed malignant or accelerated hypertension) is referred to as a 'hypertensive crisis', as blood pressure at this level confers a high risk of complications. People with blood pressures in this range may have no symptoms, but are more likely to report headaches (22% of cases) and dizziness than the general population.

Other symptoms accompanying a hypertensive crisis may include visual deterioration or breathlessness due to heart failure or a general feeling of malaise due to renal (kidney) failure. Most people with a hypertensive crisis are known to have elevated blood pressure, but additional triggers may have led to a sudden rise. A 'hypertensive emergency' is diagnosed when there is evidence of direct damage to one or more organs as a result of severely elevated blood pressure greater than 180 systolic or 120 diastolic.

Chest pain may indicate heart muscle damage (which may progress to the tearing of the inner wall of the aorta, the largest artery in the human body. Breathlessness, coughing, and the expectoration of blood-stained sputum are characteristic signs of pulmonary oedema, the swelling of lung tissue due to failure of the heart to adequately pump blood from the lungs into the arteries. Rapid deterioration of kidney function and destruction of blood cells may also occur. In these situations, rapid reduction of the blood pressure is urgently needed in order to stop organ damage. In contrast there is no evidence that blood pressure needs to be lowered rapidly in hypertensive urgencies where there is no evidence of organ damage. Aggressive reduction of blood pressure is not without risks. Use of oral medications to lower the blood pressure gradually is the best.

Pregnancy

Hypertension occurs in approximately 8–10% of pregnancies. Two blood pressure measurements six hours apart of greater than 140/90 mm Hg is considered to be indicative of hypertension in pregnancy. Most women with hypertension in pregnancy have pre-existing primary hypertension, but high blood pressure in pregnancy may be the first sign of pre-eclampsia, a serious condition of the second half of pregnancy.

Pre-eclampsia is characterised by increased blood pressure and the presence of protein in the urine. It occurs in about 5% of pregnancies and is responsible for approximately 16% of all maternal deaths globally. Pre-eclampsia also doubles the risk of perinatal mortality. Usually there are no symptoms in pre-eclampsia and it is detected by routine screening.

When symptoms of pre-eclampsia occur the most common are headache, visual disturbance, vomiting, epigastric pain, and oedema. Pre-eclampsia can occasionally progress to a life-threatening condition called eclampsia, which is a hypertensive emergency and has several serious complications including:

* vision loss,

* cerebral oedema,

* seizures or convulsions,

* kidney failure,

* pulmonary or chest oedema,

* disseminated intravascular coagulation (a blood clotting disorder).

Children

If you feel that your child is not thriving as it should, the cause could be hypertension. And this, as in adults, can possibly lead to:

Seizures,

Irritability,

lack of energy,

Difficulty in breathing can be associated with

hypertension in young infants.

In older infants and children::

headaches,

unexplained irritability,

fatigue,

blurred vision,

Nose bleeds,

facial paralysis.

Primary hypertension

Primary hypertension is the most common form of hypertension, accounting for 90–95% of all cases of hypertension. In almost all contemporary societies, blood pressure rises with ageing and the risk of becoming hypertensive in later life is considerable.

Hypertension results from a complex interaction of genes and environmental factors. Numerous common genetic variants with small effects on blood pressure have been identified as well as some rare genetic variants with large effects on blood pressure but the genetic basis of hypertension is still poorly understood.

More to the point, several environmental factors influence blood pressure.

Lifestyle factors that lower blood pressure include:

* reduced dietary salt intake,

* increased consumption of fruits

* low amounts of fat products

To these, we shall return.

Stress appears to play a minor role with specific relaxation techniques not supported by the evidence. The possible role of other factors such as caffeine consumption, and vitamin D deficiency are less clear cut. Insulin resistance, which is common in obesity and is a component of syndrome X (or the metabolic syndrome), is also thought to contribute to hypertension.

Recent studies have also implicated events in early life (for example low birth weight, maternal smoking and lack of breast feeding) as risk factors for adult hypertension, although the mechanisms linking these exposures to adult hypertension remain obscure.

Secondary hypertension

Secondary hypertension results from an identifiable cause. Renal (kidney) disease is the most common secondary cause of hypertension. Hypertension can also be caused by endocrine conditions, such as obesity, lack of sleep or irregular sleep patterns, sleep apnoea, and the physical changes during pregnancy.

Pulse pressure (the difference between systolic and diastolic blood pressure) is frequently increased in older people with hypertension. This can mean that systolic pressure is abnormally high, but diastolic pressure may be normal or low — a condition termed isolated systolic hypertension. The high pulse pressure in elderly people with hypertension or isolated systolic hypertension is explained by increased hardness of the arteries, which typically accompanies ageing and may be exacerbated by high blood pressure.

Many mechanisms have been proposed to account for the rise. Most evidence implicates either disturbances in renal (kidney) salt and water handling or abnormalities of the sympathetic nervous system. These mechanisms are not mutually exclusive and it is likely that both contribute to some extent in most cases of hypertension.

Diagnosis

Hypertension is diagnosed on the basis of a persistent high blood pressure. Traditionally, the British National Institute of Clinical Excellence recommends three separate sphygmomanometer (or blood pressure machine) measurements at monthly intervals. The American Heart Association recommends at least three measurements on at least two separate health care visits. An exception to this is those people with very high blood pressure readings especially when there is poor organ function. Initial assessment of the hypertensive people should include a complete history and physical examination. With the availability of 24-hour blood pressure monitors and home blood pressure machines, the importance of not wrongly diagnosing those who have white coat hypertension has led to a change in protocols. In the United Kingdom, current best practice is to follow up a single raised clinic reading with ambulatory measurement, or less ideally with home blood pressure monitoring over the course of 7 days.

Pseudo-hypertension in the elderly or non-compressibility artery syndrome may also require consideration. This condition is believed to be due to calcification of the arteries resulting in abnormally high blood pressure readings with a blood pressure cuff while intra-arterial measurements of blood pressure are normal.

Once the diagnosis of hypertension has been made, physicians will attempt to identify the underlying cause based on risk factors and other symptoms, if present. Secondary hypertension is more common in pre-adolescent children, with most cases caused by renal disease. Primary or essential hypertension is more common in adolescents and has multiple risk factors, including obesity and a family history of hypertension.

Laboratory tests can also be performed to identify possible causes of secondary hypertension, and to determine whether hypertension has caused damage to the heart, eyes, and kidneys. Additiona tests for diabetes and high cholesterol levels are usually performed because these conditions are additional risk factors for the development of heart disease and may require treatment.

Serum creatinine is measured to assess for the presence of kidney disease, which can be either the cause or the result of hypertension. Serum creatinine alone may overestimate glomerular filtration rate and recent guidelines advocate the use of predictive equations such as the Modification of Diet in Renal Disease (MDRD) formula to estimate glomerular filtration rate (eGFR) can also provide a baseline measurement of kidney function that can be used to monitor for side effects of certain anti-hypertensive drugs on kidney function. Additionally, testing of urine samples for protein is used as a secondary indicator of kidney disease. Electro-cardiogram (ECG) testing is done to check for evidence that the heart is under strain from high blood pressure. It may also show whether

17

there is thickening of the heart muscle or whether the heart has experienced a prior minor disturbance such as a silent heart attack. A chest X-ray or an echocardiogram may also be performed to look for signs of heart enlargement or damage to the heart.

In people aged 18 years or older hypertension is defined as a systolic and/or a diastolic blood pressure measurement consistently higher than an accepted normal value (currently 139 mmHg systolic, 89 mmHg diastolic.

Children

Hypertension in the newly-born is rare, occurring in around 0.2 to 3% of neonates, and blood pressure is not measured routinely in the healthy new-born. Hypertension is more common in high risk new-born children. A variety of factors, such as birth weight needs to be taken into account when deciding if a blood pressure is normal in a neonate.

Hypertension occurs quite commonly in children over the age of 3 years and adolescents (2-9% depending on age, sex and ethnicity) and is associated with long term risks of ill-health. Blood pressure rises with age in childhood and, in children, hypertension is defined as an average systolic or diastolic blood pressure on three or more occasions equal or higher than the 95th percentile appropriate for the sex, age and height of the child. High blood pressure must be confirmed on repeated visits however before characterizing a child as having hypertension. Pre-hypertension in children has been defined as average systolic or diastolic blood pressure that is greater than or equal to the 90th percentile, but less than the 95th percentile. In adolescents, it has been proposed that hypertension and pre-hypertension are diagnosed and classified using the same criteria as in adults.

The value of routine screening for hypertension in children over the age of 3 years is a matter for debate. In 2004 the National High Blood Pressure Education Program recommended that children aged 3 years and older have blood pressure measurement at least once at every health care visit. The National Heart, Lung, Blood Institute and American Academy of Pediatrics made a similar recommendation. However, the American Academy of Family Physicians support the view of the U.S. preventive Services Task Force that evidence is insufficient to determine the balance of benefits and harms of screening for hypertension in children and adolescents who do not have symptoms.

Prevention

Much of the disease burden of high blood pressure is experienced by people who are not labelled as hypertensive. Consequently, population strategies are required to reduce the consequences of high blood pressure and reduce the need for anti-hypertensive drug therapy. Lifestyle changes are recommended to lower blood pressure, before starting drug therapy.

The British Hypertension Society guidelines propose the following lifestyle changes consistent with those outlined by the US National High BP Education Program for the primary prevention of hypertension:

* maintain normal body weight for adults;

* reduce dietary sodium;

* engage in regular aerobic physical activity such as brisk walking;

* limit alcohol consumption to no more than 3 units/day in men and no more than 2 units/day in women;

* consume a diet rich in fruit and vegetables;

Effective lifestyle modification may lower blood pressure as much as medication. Combinations of two or more lifestyle modifications can achieve even better results.

Medication

Several classes of medications, collectively referred to as anti-hypertensive drugs, are currently available for treating hypertension. Use should take into account the person's cardiovascular risk (including risk of myocardial infarction and stroke) as well as blood pressure readings, in order to gain a more accurate picture of the person's cardiovascular profile. Evidence in those with mild hypertension and no other health problems does not support a reduction in the risk of death or rate of health complications from medication treatment. Medications are not, however, recommended for people with pre-hypertension or high normal blood pressure.

If drug treatment is initiated, it is recommended that the physician not only monitor for response to treatment but also assess any side effects resulting from the medication. Reduction of the blood pressure by 5 mmHg can decrease the risk of stroke by 34%, of ischaemic heart disease by 21%, and reduce the likelihood of dementia, heart failure, and mortality from cardiovascular disease. For most people, recommendations are to reduce blood pressure to less than or equal to somewhere between 140/90 to 160/100. Attempting to achieve lower levels have not been shown to improve outcomes, while there is evidence that it increases side effects. In those with diabetes or kidney disease some recommend levels below 120/80; however, evidence does not support these lower levels. If the blood pressure goal is not met, a change in treatment should be made.

The best first line agent is disputed. United States guidelines support prescribing a low dose thiazide-based diuretic as first line treatment. UK guidelines emphasise calcium channel blockers for people over the age of 55 years or if of African or Caribbean family origin, with angiotensin converting enzyme inhibitors (ACE-I) used as the first line for younger people. In Japan starting with any one of six classes of medications - including: CCB, ACEI/ARB, thiazide diuretics - beta-blockers and alpha-blockers are deemed reasonable, while in Canada and Europe all of these except alpha-blockers are recommended as options.

Drug combinations

The majority of people require more than one drug to control their hypertension. In those with a systolic blood pressure greater than 160 or a diastolic blood pressure greater than 100 the American Heart Association recommends starting both a thiazide and an ACEI, ARB or CCB. An ACEI and CCB combination can be used as well. There are many combinations, which will not interest the general reader for whom this book is mainly intended. There are also several unacceptable combinations. As a general rule, pills such as ibuprofen should be avoided whenever possible due to a high risk of acute renal (kidney) failure. The combination is known colloquially as a triple whammy in the Australian health industry. Tablets containing fixed combinations of two classes of drugs are available and while convenient for the people, may be best reserved for those who have been established on the individual components.

Elderly people

Treating moderate to severe hypertension decreases death rates and cardiovascular morbidity and mortality in people aged 60 and older. There are limited studies of people over 80 years old but a recent review concluded that anti-hypertensive treatment reduced cardiovascular deaths and disease, but did not significantly reduce total death rates, nor should we have expected that IT would.

The recommended Blood Pressure goal is advised as 150/90 with thiazide diuretic, CCB, ACEI, or ARB being the first line medication in the United States. In the United Kingdom guidelines, calcium-channel blockers are advocated as first line with targets of clinic readings lower than 150/90, or 145/85 on ambulatory or home blood pressure readings.

Resistant hypertension

Resistant hypertension is defined as hypertension that remains above goal blood pressure in spite of using, at once, three anti-hypertensive agents belonging to different drug classes. Guidelines for treating resistant hypertension have been published in the UK and US. It has been proposed that a proportion of resistant hypertension may be the result of chronic high activity of the autonomic nervous system; this concept is known as 'neurogenic hypertension'. Low adherence to treatment is an important cause of resistant hypertension.

Children

Rates of high blood pressure in children and adolescents have increased in the last 20 years in developed countries alone. Most childhood hypertension, particularly in pre-adolescents, is secondary to an underlying disorder. Aside from obesity, kidney disease is the most common cause of hypertension in children. (60–70%). Adolescents usually have primary or essential hypertension, which accounts for 85–95% of cases.

The first line of treatment for hypertension is identical to the recommended preventive lifestyle changes and includes dietary changes, physical exercise, and weight loss. These have all been shown to significantly reduce blood pressure in people with hypertension. Their potential effectiveness is similar to using a single medication. If hypertension is high enough to justify immediate use of medication, lifestyle changes are still recommended in conjunction with medication.

Dietary change such as a low salt intake are beneficial. A long term (more than 4 weeks) low sodium diet is effective in reducing blood pressure, both in people with hypertension and in people with normal blood pressure. Also, the DASH diet, a diet rich in nuts, whole grains, fish, poultry, fruits and vegetables lowers blood pressure. A major feature of the plan is limiting intake of sodium, although the diet is also rich in potassium, magnesium, calcium, as well as protein.

Some programs, aimed to reduce psychological stress, such as transcendental meditation may be reasonable additions to other treatment. However techniques such as yoga, relaxation and other forms of meditation do not appear to reduce blood pressure, and, of the techniques with supportive evidence, there is limited information on whether the modest reduction in blood pressure results in prevention of cardiovascular disease.

Several exercise regimes—including isometric resistance exercise, aerobic exercise, resistance exercise and device-guided breathing—may be useful in reducing blood pressure.

Dr Mary-Beth can only be contacted through the publisher. Even then, she cannot promise to give advice. However she is always ready to discuss problems of a medical nature.

The doctor is far too busy with her daily hospital duties and her limited private practice to have any time to spare for time-wasters.